CONTENTS

INTRODUCTION

Welcome to the Fatty Liver Diet Cookbook, a burst of flavors and nourishment crafted to guide you on a transformative journey towards optimal liver health and well-being. Within these pages, you'll discover a world of culinary possibilities designed to demystify the complexities of managing fatty liver disease while embracing the joy of delicious and nutrient-rich meals.

Your journey begins here, as we explore the intricate connection between the food you enjoy and the health of your liver. Fatty liver disease is a condition that demands attention, understanding, and action, and this cookbook is your trusted companion on this path to vitality.

In the chapters that follow, you'll delve into a wealth of knowledge, burst-worthy recipes, and practical strategies that empower you to make informed choices for your health. From the principles of a balanced diet and the art of mindful eating to the magic of incorporating liver-supportive ingredients into your meals, each turn of the page invites you to embark on a culinary adventure that not only supports your liver but also delights your taste buds.

Navigating the realm of nutrition doesn't have to be overwhelming. That's why this cookbook is here to serve as a burst of clarity, a resource that not only provides delicious recipes but also equips you with the tools to understand the nutritional value of each dish. As you embark on this journey, you'll find that every recipe is a burst of creativity, a canvas on which you can paint your health goals, one vibrant ingredient at a time.

Beyond the kitchen, this cookbook recognizes the holistic nature of well-being. You'll explore the significance of regular exercise, the art of stress reduction, the importance of quality sleep, and how to seek support from medical professionals. Each of these elements contributes to the symphony of a healthy lifestyle, creating a harmonious burst of vitality that radiates from within.

Your journey through the Fatty Liver Diet Cookbook is an invitation to savor each moment, celebrate every step of progress, and embrace the potential for transformation. As you experiment with flavors, adapt your habits, and embrace new approaches to nourishment, may you find inspiration in the burst of colors, aromas, and tastes that unfold on your plate.

Whether you're embarking on this journey to support your own liver health or are here as a source of guidance for a loved one, this cookbook is a testament to the power of nourishing choices. It's a burst of empowerment—an embodiment of the notion that through mindful eating, informed decisions, and a dash of culinary creativity, you hold the key to your own well-being.

So, welcome to the Fatty Liver Diet Cookbook, a burst of knowledge, a burst of flavor, and a burst of transformation. Let's embark on this journey together, as we celebrate the burst-worthy potential of food to heal, nurture, and revitalize. Your path to a healthier you begins now.

CHAPTER ONE

*Introduction to Fatty Liver
and Diet Management*

Understanding Fatty Liver Disease

Fatty liver disease, a term encompassing non-alcoholic fatty liver disease (NAFLD) and its more advanced form non-alcoholic steatohepatitis (NASH), is a prevalent yet perplexing health condition that has become a burgeoning concern worldwide. This condition is characterized by an excessive accumulation of fat in liver cells, leading to impairment in liver function and potential long-term health implications. The enigmatic nature of fatty liver disease lies in its subtle progression, often remaining asymptomatic until significant damage has occurred. Bursting onto the medical scene as a major public health issue, fatty liver disease is shrouded in mystery due to its multifaceted causative factors and varying degrees of severity.

The intricate dance of genetic predisposition, metabolic disruptions, and lifestyle choices choreographs the onset of fatty liver disease. While obesity and insulin resistance perform a duet in promoting fat buildup in the liver, the harmony is further disrupted by factors such as sedentary lifestyles, poor dietary habits, and even genetic variations. Unraveling the precise interplay between these elements has baffled researchers and clinicians alike, leading to the perplexity surrounding its diagnosis and treatment. The liver's central role in metabolic regulation adds to the mystique, as the organ's intricate tasks are disrupted by the accumulation of excess fat, potentially leading to inflammation and scarring.

Importance of Diet in Managing Fatty Liver

Amidst the complexity of fatty liver disease, the spotlight shines brightly on the importance of diet as a key player in its management. A diet rich in nutrients and mindful of caloric intake can be a beacon of hope in mitigating the progression of this enigmatic condition. Bursting with potential, dietary interventions can contribute significantly to reducing fat accumulation in the liver, thereby addressing one of the core issues of the disease. To demystify this aspect, it's crucial to break down several dietary factors that come into play.

- Reduced Sugar Intake: Excessive sugar consumption, especially in the form of fructose, can contribute to liver fat accumulation. High fructose corn syrup, commonly found in sugary beverages and processed foods, can be particularly burdensome for the liver. Thus, curbing added sugars and opting for natural sources of sweetness can be a perplexingly effective strategy.
- Healthy Fats: While reducing fat intake might seem like a logical step, the type of fat matters significantly. Healthy fats such as those found in avocados, nuts, and fatty fish burst forth as allies in managing fatty liver. These fats offer a paradoxical solution, as they promote a sense of

fullness while potentially aiding in reducing liver fat accumulation.

- Complex Carbohydrates: The conundrum of carbohydrates lies in their complexity. Opting for whole grains and fiber-rich carbohydrates instead of refined options can assist in managing insulin levels, which in turn might help prevent excessive fat buildup in the liver.

- Portion Control: The burstiness of portion control cannot be overstated. Eating in moderation, regardless of the nutritional quality of the food, is a powerful approach to managing weight and subsequently alleviating fatty liver disease. Understanding portion sizes can be perplexing, but tools like mindful eating and portion-awareness can aid in unraveling this dietary riddle.

How This Cookbook Can Help

In the midst of this health maze, a cookbook specifically designed to cater to the needs of individuals dealing with fatty liver disease can emerge as a guiding light. This cookbook, enriched with culinary creativity and nutritional wisdom, can play a vital role in demystifying the perplexities of managing this condition through diet.

- Tailored Recipes: This cookbook can offer a treasure trove of recipes tailored to the dietary requirements of individuals with fatty liver disease. Bursting with flavors and textures, these recipes can include a variety of nutrient-rich ingredients that support liver health while ensuring a satisfying gastronomic experience.

- Educational Content: Beyond just recipes, the cookbook can burst forth with educational content. From deciphering the nuances of nutrient labels to providing insightful explanations about the roles of various food components, this cookbook can empower individuals to make informed dietary decisions that align with their health goals.
- Meal Planning Strategies: One of the perplexities individuals face is the challenge of creating well-balanced meals that support liver health. This cookbook can unveil meal planning strategies, helping individuals put together meals that are not only delicious but also contribute positively to their liver function.
- Lifestyle Integration: The cookbook can transcend its pages and guide users in integrating healthy dietary choices into their lifestyles. Bursting beyond the confines of recipes, it can offer tips on grocery shopping, kitchen organization, and even stress management, all of which play a role in managing fatty liver disease.

In conclusion, the perplexing nature of fatty liver disease, intertwined with its multifaceted causative factors and enigmatic progression, necessitates a holistic approach to management. Diet, bursting forth as a pivotal player in this narrative, offers the potential to address the core issue of fat accumulation in the liver. A cookbook tailored to the needs of individuals dealing with fatty liver disease can serve as a guiding light, offering not only delicious recipes but also educational content and lifestyle strategies to demystify the journey toward liver health. Through understanding the intricacies of the disease and embracing a dietary revolution, individuals can navigate this health challenge with empowered perseverance.

CHAPTER TWO

Fatty Liver Explained

Different Types of Fatty Liver Disease

Fatty liver disease isn't a monolithic condition; rather, it's a family of liver disorders that involve the accumulation of fat within liver cells. The two main types are non-alcoholic fatty liver disease (NAFLD) and alcoholic fatty liver disease. Each type presents its own unique perplexities, adding to the overall complexity of the condition.

- Non-Alcoholic Fatty Liver Disease (NAFLD): This is the most common form of fatty liver disease and is characterized by excess fat in the liver that isn't due to alcohol consumption. It encompasses a spectrum of conditions, ranging from simple steatosis (fat accumulation) to non-alcoholic steatohepatitis (NASH), which involves inflammation and potential scarring of the liver tissue.

- Alcoholic Fatty Liver Disease: As the name suggests, this type of fatty liver disease is directly linked to excessive alcohol consumption. It occurs due to the toxic effects of alcohol on the liver, leading to the accumulation of fat. While moderate alcohol consumption might not necessarily cause this condition, heavy drinking over time can significantly impact liver function.

Causes and Risk Factors

The causes and risk factors behind fatty liver disease are a jigsaw puzzle with multiple intricate pieces that interact in complex ways. Understanding the individual pieces can help demystify the overall picture of this perplexing condition.

- Genetics: Genetic factors play a role in determining an individual's susceptibility to developing fatty liver disease. Certain genetic variations can influence how the body processes fats and carbohydrates, potentially contributing to fat accumulation in the liver.
- Obesity and Insulin Resistance: These twin culprits are strongly linked to fatty liver disease. Excess weight, particularly around the abdominal area, and insulin resistance can promote the accumulation of fat in the liver cells.
- Dietary Factors: Diets high in added sugars, refined carbohydrates, and unhealthy fats can contribute to the development of fatty liver disease. The burstiness of these dietary choices can lead to metabolic disruptions and increased fat storage in the liver.
- Lifestyle Choices: Sedentary lifestyles and lack of physical activity can be significant risk factors. Exercise helps regulate insulin sensitivity and aids in weight management, both of which are crucial for preventing fatty liver disease.

Symptoms and Diagnosis

The symptoms of fatty liver disease are often elusive, leading to a sense of mystery and perplexity. It's not uncommon for individuals to remain asymptomatic until the disease has progressed significantly. However, some potential symptoms and diagnostic approaches can shed light on the coDiagnosi

Symptoms: In the early stages, fatty liver disease might not cause noticeable symptoms. As the disease progresses, individuals might experience fatigue, weakness, discomfort in the upper right abdomen, or unexplained weight loss. These symptoms can be vague and easily mistaken for other health issues.

Diagnostic Tools: Various diagnostic tools contribute to unraveling the enigma of fatty liver disease. Imaging studies like ultrasound, CT scans, and MRI can visualize fat accumulation in the liver. However, a liver biopsy is the gold standard for confirming the diagnosis and assessing the degree of inflammation and scarring.

Blood Tests: Blood tests can provide valuable insights into liver function. Elevated levels of liver enzymes, such as alanine transaminase (ALT) and aspartate transaminase (AST), can indicate liver damage. Additionally, other markers like gamma-glutamyl transferase (GGT) and the presence of certain proteins can contribute to the diagnostic puzzle.

Fibrosis Assessment: As fatty liver disease progresses, it can lead to fibrosis (scarring) of the liver tissue, which is a serious complication. Non-invasive methods like FibroScan and blood tests that measure fibrosis-related markers can help assess the extent of liver damage without the need for a biopsy.

In conclusion, the complexity of fatty liver disease extends beyond its classification into different types. The multifaceted causative factors, encompassing genetics, lifestyle choices, and dietary habits, create a perplexing web that contributes to its development. Symptom manifestation and diagnosis add another layer of mystery, as the disease can remain hidden until advanced stages. Unraveling these complexities requires a combination of medical expertise, diagnostic tools, and a comprehensive understanding of the puzzle pieces that contribute to the enigma of fatty liver disease.

CHAPTER THREE

The Foundations of a Fatty Liver-Friendly Diet

Principles of a Balanced Diet for Liver Health

Maintaining a balanced diet is a cornerstone in the perplexing puzzle of promoting liver health. The principles of a balanced diet for liver health are geared towards providing essential nutrients while minimizing factors that contribute to fat accumulation and inflammation in the liver. Bursting with wisdom, these principles aim to demystify the journey towards a healthier liver.

- Moderation: The principle of moderation takes center stage. Balancing portion sizes and caloric intake is essential to prevent overloading the liver with excess energy. Moderation extends to all food groups, ensuring a varied and well-rounded diet.
- Variety: Bursting forth with nutrients, a variety of foods ensures the intake of a wide range of essential vitamins, minerals, and phytochemicals. Different foods offer different liver-supportive compounds, making dietary diversity a key principle.
- Whole Foods: Choosing whole, unprocessed foods provides the body with essential nutrients without the burden of added sugars, unhealthy

fats, and artificial additives. Whole foods burst forth with nutrients that nourish the liver and support its function.

- Hydration: Staying hydrated is essential for liver health. Water aids in digestion, detoxification, and overall bodily functions. Hydration is like a burst of vitality for the liver, helping it perform its tasks efficiently.

Nutrients to Focus On: Fiber, Antioxidants, Healthy Fats, etc.

Fiber: Dietary fiber, found in fruits, vegetables, whole grains, and legumes, is a burst of digestive support. It aids in regular bowel movements, preventing constipation and promoting a healthy gut microbiome, which indirectly impacts liver health.

- Antioxidants: Colorful fruits and vegetables burst with antioxidants like vitamins C and E, which help combat oxidative stress and inflammation in the liver. These nutrients protect liver cells from damage and support their optimal function.
- Healthy Fats: Incorporating healthy fats from sources like avocados, nuts, seeds, and fatty fish is essential. These fats provide omega-3 fatty acids that have anti-inflammatory properties, benefiting liver health and overall well-being.
- Lean Proteins: Including lean sources of protein, such as poultry, fish, beans, and tofu, provides amino acids necessary for cell repair and maintenance. These proteins contribute to the burst of vitality needed for healthy liver function.
- Vitamins and Minerals: Nutrients like vitamin

D, vitamin B complex, zinc, and magnesium play important roles in liver health. Bursting with significance, they support various metabolic processes and aid in detoxification.

Foods to Avoid: High Sugar, Processed Foods, Alcohol, etc.

- High Sugar Foods: Foods and beverages laden with added sugars cause a burst of detrimental effects on the liver. Excess sugar leads to fat accumulation and insulin resistance, both of which contribute to fatty liver disease.
- Processed Foods: Highly processed foods often burst forth with unhealthy fats, excess sodium, and artificial additives. These burden the liver and contribute to inflammation, impairing its function over time.
- Trans Fats: Trans fats, commonly found in fried and processed foods, are perplexing foes for liver health. They promote inflammation and can contribute to the development of fatty liver disease.
- Alcohol: The liver's relationship with alcohol is complicated. Excessive alcohol consumption is directly linked to alcoholic fatty liver disease and can lead to more severe liver conditions. Bursting with potential harm, alcohol should be consumed in moderation, if at all.
- Highly Processed Meats: Processed meats, such as sausages, hot dogs, and deli meats, are often high in sodium, preservatives, and unhealthy fats. These foods can contribute to liver inflammation and overall health issues.

In conclusion, understanding the principles of a balanced diet for liver health is paramount to unraveling the perplexities of maintaining a healthy liver. Prioritizing moderation, variety, and whole foods while focusing on nutrients like fiber, antioxidants, and healthy fats is key. Simultaneously, avoiding high sugar foods, processed options, trans fats, alcohol, and highly processed meats contributes to the puzzle of supporting liver health. By following these principles and making mindful dietary choices, individuals can burst forth with positive impacts on their liver health and overall well-being.

CHAPTER FOUR

Kitchen Staples for Liver Health

Essential Ingredients for a Fatty Liver Diet

Crafting a fatty liver diet that supports liver health involves selecting essential ingredients that provide necessary nutrients while minimizing factors that contribute to fat accumulation and inflammation. These ingredients, bursting with potential, form the foundation of a diet aimed at demystifying the complexities of managing fatty liver disease.

Stocking Up on Whole Grains, Lean Proteins, and Fresh Produce

- Whole Grains: Bursting with fiber, vitamins, and minerals, whole grains like brown rice, quinoa, whole wheat pasta, and oats are essential. They promote stable blood sugar levels and support digestive health, indirectly aiding liver function.
- Lean Proteins: Incorporating lean sources of protein is pivotal. Skinless poultry, fish, tofu, tempeh, legumes, and beans provide essential amino acids for cell repair and immune function without the burden of excessive unhealthy fats.
- Fresh Produce: Colorful fruits and vegetables burst forth with antioxidants, vitamins, and

minerals that support liver health. Berries, leafy greens, cruciferous vegetables, and citrus fruits provide a burst of beneficial nutrients.

Healthy Cooking Oils and Herbs/Spices that Support Liver Function

- Healthy Cooking Oils: Opting for healthy cooking oils like olive oil, avocado oil, and coconut oil is crucial. These oils burst with heart-healthy fats and antioxidants that support liver health and protect against inflammation.
- Turmeric: Bursting with the active compound curcumin, turmeric has potent anti-inflammatory and antioxidant properties. Adding this spice to dishes can benefit liver function and help reduce inflammation.
- Garlic: Garlic is not only bursting with flavor but also contains compounds that support liver detoxification processes. It can be used as a seasoning in various dishes to enhance liver health.
- Ginger: Ginger is known for its anti-inflammatory and antioxidant properties. Incorporating it into meals or preparing ginger tea can provide a burst of benefits for liver health.
- Cinnamon: Cinnamon bursts with natural sweetness and is believed to improve insulin sensitivity. This spice can help regulate blood sugar levels, which is important for managing fatty liver disease.

Other Essential Ingredients

- Nuts and Seeds: Almonds, walnuts, chia seeds, and flaxseeds are rich in healthy fats, fiber, and antioxidants. They can be sprinkled on salads, yogurt, or oatmeal for a burst of nutrients.
- Avocado: Avocado is a creamy and nutritious ingredient bursting with healthy monounsaturated fats. It can be used in salads, sandwiches, or as a spread to provide a burst of flavor and nutrition.
- Low-Fat Dairy or Dairy Alternatives: Including low-fat dairy or dairy alternatives like almond milk or Greek yogurt provides a source of calcium and protein while minimizing saturated fat intake.
- Herbal Teas: Herbal teas like green tea and dandelion tea offer a burst of antioxidants that support liver health. They can be enjoyed as a soothing beverage throughout the day.
- Citrus Fruits: Bursting with vitamin C, citrus fruits like oranges, grapefruits, and lemons support the body's detoxification processes and provide a refreshing burst of flavor.

In conclusion, essential ingredients for a fatty liver diet burst forth with nutrient-rich options that support liver health. Stocking up on whole grains, lean proteins, and fresh produce ensures a balanced and nourishing diet. Healthy cooking oils, along with liver-supporting herbs and spices, add bursts of flavor and benefits. By incorporating these essential ingredients into daily meals, individuals can unravel the perplexities of managing fatty liver disease and promote overall well-being.

CHAPTER FIVE

Breakfasts to Kickstart Your Day

Nutrient-rich Smoothies and Juices

Description of the Meal:

Indulge in the vibrant goodness of our nutrient-rich smoothies and juices that will invigorate your senses and boost your energy levels. Whether you're looking for a refreshing morning pick-me-up or a post-workout revitalization, these drinks are packed with vitamins, minerals, and antioxidants to keep you feeling your best.

Ingredients:

- 1 ripe banana, peeled and sliced
- 1 cup mixed berries (strawberries, blueberries, raspberries)
- 1 cup spinach leaves
- 1/2 avocado, pitted and scooped
- 1 tablespoon chia seeds
- 1 cup almond milk
- 1 tablespoon honey
- Ice cubes

Instructions:

- In a blender, combine the banana, mixed berries, spinach, avocado, chia seeds, almond milk, and honey.

- Blend on high until smooth and creamy, adding ice cubes as desired for thickness.
- Pour into glasses and garnish with additional berries or a sprinkle of chia seeds if desired.
- Serve immediately and enjoy the refreshing burst of flavors and nutrients.

Nutritional Information:

- Calories: 250
- Protein: 5g
- Carbohydrates: 40g
- Fiber: 9g
- Fat: 9g
- Vitamins: A, C, K
- Minerals: Potassium, Calcium, Iron

Fiber-packed Oatmeal Variations
Description of the Meal:

Experience the heartiness and satisfaction of our fiber-packed oatmeal variations. These warm and comforting bowls are not only delicious but also rich in dietary fiber, promoting healthy digestion and keeping you full for longer.

Ingredients:

- 1 cup rolled oats
- 2 cups water or milk of your choice
- 1 sliced banana
- 1/4 cup chopped nuts (almonds, walnuts, or pecans)
- 1 tablespoon chia seeds
- 1/2 teaspoon cinnamon
- 1/4 cup mixed dried fruits (raisins, cranberries,

apricots)
- 1 tablespoon honey or maple syrup

Instructions:

- In a saucepan, bring the water or milk to a boil, then add the rolled oats.
- Reduce the heat to a simmer and cook the oats, stirring occasionally, until they reach your desired consistency.
- Remove from heat and stir in the sliced banana, chopped nuts, chia seeds, cinnamon, and mixed dried fruits.
- Drizzle with honey or maple syrup for sweetness.
- Serve warm in bowls and savor the comforting textures and flavors.

Nutritional Information:

- Calories: 350
- Protein: 8g
- Carbohydrates: 55g
- Fiber: 10g
- Fat: 12g
- Vitamins: B6
- Minerals: Magnesium, Phosphorus, Manganese

Egg-based Dishes with a Focus on Veggies
Description of the Meal:

Dive into the world of egg-based dishes with a twist! Our creations put the spotlight on veggies, delivering a colorful and nutritious culinary experience. From fluffy omelets to savory scrambles, these meals will delight your taste buds and nourish your body.

Ingredients:

- 2 eggs
- 1/4 cup diced bell peppers (assorted colors)
- 1/4 cup chopped spinach
- 1/4 cup diced tomatoes
- 2 tablespoons diced onion
- 1/4 cup grated cheese (cheddar, mozzarella, or feta)
- Salt and pepper to taste
- Fresh herbs (parsley, chives) for garnish

Instructions:

- In a bowl, whisk the eggs and season with salt and pepper.
- Heat a non-stick skillet over medium heat and add a drizzle of oil.
- Sauté the diced bell peppers, chopped spinach, diced tomatoes, and diced onion until softened.
- Pour the whisked eggs over the sautéed veggies and cook until the edges start to set.
- Sprinkle the grated cheese on one half of the omelet and fold the other half over it.
- Cook for another minute until the cheese melts and the eggs are fully set.
- Slide the omelet onto a plate, garnish with fresh herbs, and serve with whole-grain toast.

Nutritional Information:

- Calories: 280
- Protein: 18g
- Carbohydrates: 10g
- Fiber: 2g
- Fat: 20g
- Vitamins: A, C, D
- Minerals: Calcium, Iron, Potassium

Lunches for Sustained Energy
Fresh and Hearty Salads
Description of the Meal:

Embrace the vibrant flavors and textures of our fresh and hearty salads that are a feast for both your eyes and your taste buds. Bursting with colors, these nutrient-packed salads combine crisp vegetables, wholesome grains, and delectable dressings to create a satisfying and healthful dining experience.

Ingredients:

- 2 cups mixed salad greens (lettuce, spinach, arugula)
- 1 cup cherry tomatoes, halved
- 1 cucumber, sliced
- 1/2 cup diced bell peppers (assorted colors)
- 1/4 red onion, thinly sliced
- 1/2 cup cooked quinoa
- 1/4 cup feta cheese, crumbled
- 1/4 cup toasted nuts (walnuts, almonds, or pine nuts)
- Balsamic vinaigrette dressing

Instructions:

- In a large bowl, combine the mixed salad greens, cherry tomatoes, cucumber, diced bell peppers, and red onion.
- Add the cooked quinoa and crumbled feta cheese to the salad.
- Drizzle with your favorite balsamic vinaigrette dressing and toss to combine.
- Top the salad with toasted nuts for added crunch

and flavor.
- Serve immediately and relish the refreshing medley of ingredients.

Nutritional Information:

- Calories: 320
- Protein: 10g
- Carbohydrates: 30g
- Fiber: 6g
- Fat: 18g
- Vitamins: A, C, K
- Minerals: Calcium, Magnesium, Potassium

Whole Grain Wraps and Sandwiche
Description of the Meal:

Delight in the convenience and wholesomeness of our whole grain wraps and sandwiches, perfect for a satisfying on-the-go meal. These creations feature a harmonious blend of lean proteins, crisp veggies, and hearty whole grains, providing a balanced and delectable dining experience.

Ingredients:

- 1 whole grain wrap or bread slice
- 3 oz grilled chicken breast, sliced
- 1/4 avocado, sliced
- 1/4 cup shredded carrots
- 1/4 cup baby spinach leaves
- 2 tablespoons hummus
- Salt and pepper to taste

Instructions:

- Lay out the whole grain wrap or bread slice on a

clean surface.

- Spread a layer of hummus evenly over the wrap or bread.
- Arrange the sliced grilled chicken, avocado, shredded carrots, and baby spinach leaves on top.
- Season with a pinch of salt and pepper for flavor.
- Roll up the wrap tightly, securing it with a toothpick if needed.
- Slice the wrap in half diagonally and serve as a portable and nutritious meal.

Nutritional Information:

- Calories: 380
- Protein: 30g
- Carbohydrates: 25g
- Fiber: 8g
- Fat: 18g
- Vitamins: B6, K
- Minerals: Iron, Potassium, Zinc

Homemade Soups with Liver-Friendly Ingredients

Description of the Meal:

Nourish your body with our homemade soups featuring liver-friendly ingredients that promote well-being and vitality. These flavorful soups are crafted with care, incorporating ingredients known for their positive impact on liver health, making them a delicious way to support your body's detoxification processes.

Ingredients:

- 1 tablespoon olive oil
- 1 onion, chopped

- 2 cloves garlic, minced
- 2 carrots, diced
- 2 celery stalks, diced
- 1 cup chopped kale or spinach
- 6 cups low-sodium vegetable broth
- 1 cup diced sweet potatoes
- 1 teaspoon turmeric
- 1 teaspoon ginger, grated
- Salt and pepper to taste
- Fresh lemon juice for serving

Instructions:

- In a large pot, heat the olive oil over medium heat.
- Sauté the chopped onion and minced garlic until fragrant and translucent.
- Add the diced carrots, celery, and chopped kale or spinach. Cook for a few minutes until slightly softened.
- Pour in the low-sodium vegetable broth and add the diced sweet potatoes, turmeric, and grated ginger.
- Season with salt and pepper to taste and bring the soup to a simmer.
- Cover and let the soup simmer until the sweet potatoes are tender.
- Once cooked, use an immersion blender to puree the soup until smooth.
- Serve the soup hot, drizzled with a splash of fresh lemon juice for a zesty kick.

Nutritional Information:

- Calories: 180
- Protein: 4g
- Carbohydrates: 30g

- Fiber: 6g
- Fat: 6g
- Vitamins: A, C, K
- Minerals: Potassium, Iron, Magnesium

Wholesome Snacks for Munching
Nut and Seed Mixes
Description of the Meal:

Savor the perfect balance of crunch and flavor with our delightful nut and seed mixes. These mixes are carefully crafted to provide a wholesome blend of nutrient-dense nuts and seeds, offering a satisfying and energizing snack that's ideal for any time of the day.

Ingredients:

- 1/4 cup almonds
- 1/4 cup walnuts
- 2 tablespoons pumpkin seeds
- 2 tablespoons sunflower seeds
- 2 tablespoons dried cranberries or raisins
- 1 teaspoon cinnamon
- 1/4 teaspoon sea salt

Instructions:

- In a bowl, combine the almonds, walnuts, pumpkin seeds, sunflower seeds, and dried cranberries or raisins.
- Sprinkle the cinnamon and sea salt over the mixture.
- Toss the ingredients together until evenly distributed.
- Portion the nut and seed mix into small snack-sized bags for easy on-the-go enjoyment.

- Store in a cool, dry place to maintain freshness.

Nutritional Information:

- Calories: 220
- Protein: 7g
- Carbohydrates: 11g
- Fiber: 3g
- Fat: 18g
- Minerals: Magnesium, Zinc

Greek Yogurt Parfaits

Description of the Meal:

Indulge in the creamy goodness of our Greek yogurt parfaits, a delightful combination of protein-rich yogurt, sweet fruits, and crunchy toppings. These parfaits are not only a feast for your taste buds but also provide a dose of probiotics for gut health.

Ingredients:

- 1 cup Greek yogurt (plain or vanilla)
- 1/2 cup mixed berries (blueberries, strawberries, raspberries)
- 1/4 cup granola
- 1 tablespoon honey
- Fresh mint leaves for garnish

Instructions:

- In a glass or bowl, layer half of the Greek yogurt.
- Add a layer of mixed berries on top of the yogurt.
- Sprinkle a portion of granola over the berries.
- Drizzle with a touch of honey for sweetness.
- Repeat the layering process with the remaining yogurt, berries, and granola.

- Garnish with fresh mint leaves for a burst of freshness.
- Dive into the parfait with a spoon and enjoy the delightful combination of textures.

Nutritional Information:

- Calories: 300
- Protein: 15g
- Carbohydrates: 40g
- Fiber: 4g
- Fat: 9g
- Vitamins: C
- Minerals: Calcium

Vegetable Sticks with Healthy Dip
Description of the Meal:

Dive into a medley of colors and flavors with our vegetable sticks paired with healthy dips. These satisfying snacks offer a fun and nutritious way to enjoy an array of vitamins, minerals, and antioxidants while indulging in a variety of tasty dips.

Ingredients:

- 1 carrot, cut into sticks
- 1 cucumber, cut into sticks
- 1 bell pepper, cut into strips
- 1 celery stalk, cut into sticks
- 1 cup cherry tomatoes
- Hummus
- Greek yogurt and herb dip

Instructions:

- Arrange the carrot sticks, cucumber sticks, bell

 pepper strips, celery sticks, and cherry tomatoes on a serving platter.
- Serve alongside bowls of hummus and Greek yogurt and herb dip.
- Dip the vegetable sticks into the dips and enjoy the crisp textures and flavors.

Nutritional Information:

- Calories (with 2 tablespoons hummus and 2 tablespoons dip): 150
- Protein: 6g
- Carbohydrates: 20g
- Fiber: 7g
- Fat: 6g
- Vitamins: A, C, K
- Minerals: Potassium

Nourishing Dinners for Optimal Liver Function Lean Protein Options: Fish, Poultry, Tofu

Description of the Meal:

Discover the delectable world of lean protein with our assortment of fish, poultry, and tofu dishes. These options are tailored to satisfy your taste buds and provide essential nutrients while promoting overall health and well-being.

Ingredients:

- 6 oz grilled salmon fillet (or chicken breast/tofu)
- 1 tablespoon olive oil
- Fresh lemon juice
- Salt and pepper to taste

Instructions:

- Preheat a grill or grill pan over medium heat.

- Brush the salmon fillet (or chicken/tofu) with olive oil and season with salt and pepper.
- Grill the salmon fillet (or cook chicken/tofu) for about 3-4 minutes on each side, or until fully cooked.
- Squeeze fresh lemon juice over the cooked protein.
- Serve with your choice of roasted vegetables and a side of quinoa or brown rice-based dish.

Nutritional Information (Salmon):

- Calories: 300
- Protein: 30g
- Carbohydrates: 0g
- Fat: 20g
- Vitamins: D, B12
- Minerals: Omega-3 Fatty Acids

Roasted and Steamed Vegetable Medleys
Description of the Meal:

Experience a symphony of flavors and colors with our roasted and steamed vegetable medleys. Packed with essential vitamins, minerals, and dietary fiber, these dishes offer a delightful and healthful way to elevate your meals.

Ingredients:

- 2 cups mixed vegetables (broccoli florets, carrots, bell peppers)
- 1 tablespoon olive oil
- Salt and pepper to taste

Instructions:

For Roasted Vegetables:

- Preheat the oven to 400°F (200°C).

- Toss the mixed vegetables with olive oil, salt, and pepper.
- Spread the vegetables on a baking sheet in a single layer.
- Roast in the preheated oven for 20-25 minutes or until the vegetables are tender and slightly caramelized.

For Steamed Vegetables:

- Place a steamer basket in a pot filled with water, ensuring the water doesn't touch the bottom of the basket.
- Add the mixed vegetables to the steamer basket.
- Cover the pot and steam the vegetables over medium heat for 5-7 minutes or until they are cooked to your desired tenderness.

Nutritional Information (Roasted Vegetables):

- Calories: 100
- Carbohydrates: 10g
- Fiber: 4g
- Vitamins: A, C
- Minerals: Potassium

Quinoa and Brown Rice-Based Dishes
Description of the Meal:

Savor the nourishing goodness of quinoa and brown rice-based dishes that offer a wholesome foundation for your meals. These versatile grains provide complex carbohydrates, dietary fiber, and essential nutrients to support your active lifestyle.

Ingredients:

- 1 cup cooked quinoa
- 1 cup cooked brown rice
- 1 cup mixed sautéed vegetables (zucchini, bell peppers, onions)
- 1/4 cup chopped fresh herbs (parsley, cilantro)
- 2 tablespoons olive oil
- Lemon zest and juice
- Salt and pepper to taste

Instructions:

- In a large bowl, combine the cooked quinoa, cooked brown rice, mixed sautéed vegetables, and chopped fresh herbs.
- Drizzle olive oil over the mixture and toss to combine.
- Add lemon zest and juice for a burst of flavor.
- Season with salt and pepper to taste.
- Serve as a satisfying side dish or add lean protein (fish, poultry, tofu) for a complete meal.

Nutritional Information:

- Calories (per 1 cup serving): 300
- Protein: 8g
- Carbohydrates: 45g
- Fiber: 6g
- Fat: 10g
- Vitamins: B6, K
- Minerals: Magnesium, Manganese

Sides and Salads to Complement Your Meals
Colorful Vegetable Side Dishes
Description of the Meal:

Elevate your meal with a burst of vibrant colors and flavors from our colorful vegetable side dishes. These dishes not only add visual appeal to your plate but also provide a wealth of vitamins, minerals, and antioxidants to enhance your overall well-being.

Ingredients:

- 2 cups mixed colorful vegetables (carrots, bell peppers, broccoli, cherry tomatoes)
- 2 tablespoons olive oil
- 1 teaspoon mixed dried herbs (thyme, rosemary, oregano)
- Salt and pepper to taste

Instructions:

- Preheat the oven to 400°F (200°C).
- Toss the mixed colorful vegetables with olive oil, dried herbs, salt, and pepper.
- Spread the vegetables on a baking sheet in a single layer.
- Roast in the preheated oven for 15-20 minutes or until the vegetables are tender and slightly caramelized.
- Serve as a vibrant side dish that complements any main course.

Nutritional Information:

- Calories: 100
- Carbohydrates: 10g
- Fiber: 4g
- Vitamins: A, C
- Minerals: Potassium

Legume-Based Salad
Description of the Meal:

Indulge in the goodness of legume-based salads that combine the nourishing power of beans and lentils with an array of flavorful ingredients. These salads offer a satisfying blend of protein, fiber, and complex carbohydrates, perfect for a light and hearty meal.

Ingredients:

- 1 cup cooked chickpeas (garbanzo beans)
- 1 cup cooked black beans
- 1 cup cooked green lentils
- 1 cup diced colorful bell peppers
- 1/2 cup diced red onion
- 1/4 cup chopped fresh herbs (parsley, cilantro)
- 1/4 cup feta cheese, crumbled (optional)
- Balsamic vinaigrette dressing

Instructions:

- In a large bowl, combine the cooked chickpeas, black beans, green lentils, diced bell peppers, diced red onion, and chopped fresh herbs.
- If desired, sprinkle crumbled feta cheese over the salad.
- Drizzle balsamic vinaigrette dressing over the mixture and toss to combine.
- Serve as a protein-packed salad that's bursting with textures and flavors.

Nutritional Information:

- Calories (without feta): 350
- Protein: 20g
- Carbohydrates: 60g
- Fiber: 15g
- Fat: 5g
- Vitamins: B6, C

- Minerals: Iron, Magnesium

Fermented Foods for Gut Health
Description of the Meal:

Nurture your gut health with the goodness of fermented foods that are rich in probiotics and digestive enzymes. These foods provide a flavorful and nourishing way to support your gut microbiome and promote overall wellness.

Ingredients:

- 1 cup plain yogurt or kefir
- 1/2 cup sauerkraut
- 1/4 cup kimchi
- 1/4 cup kombucha
- Slices of whole-grain sourdough bread

Instructions:

- Serve a portion of plain yogurt or kefir in a bowl as a base.
- Arrange a side of sauerkraut and kimchi on the plate.
- Pour a glass of chilled kombucha for a refreshing fermented beverage.
- Enjoy the assortment of fermented foods along with slices of whole-grain sourdough bread.

Nutritional Information (Plain Yogurt or Kefir):

- Calories: 150
- Protein: 12g
- Carbohydrates: 15g
- Fat: 6g
- Vitamins: B12, D

- Minerals: Calcium, Probiotics

CHAPTER SIX

Satisfying Vegetarian and Vegan Options
Plant-Based Protein Sources

- Embracing a plant-based diet bursting with protein is essential for those seeking to support liver health without relying on meat. These plant-powered protein sources are not only nutrient-rich but also contribute to overall well-being.
- Legumes: Bursting with protein, fiber, and various vitamins, legumes like lentils, chickpeas, black beans, and kidney beans are versatile ingredients. They can be used in soups, salads, curries, and more.
- Tofu and Tempeh: Soy-based products like tofu and tempeh are complete sources of protein, meaning they contain all essential amino acids. Bursting with adaptability, they can be grilled, stir-fried, or added to wraps.
- Quinoa: This ancient grain is a complete protein source and is also rich in fiber and essential nutrients. Bursting with versatility, quinoa can be used as a base for salads, bowls, or even as a breakfast porridge.
- Nuts and Seeds: Almonds, walnuts, chia seeds, flaxseeds, and pumpkin seeds are bursting with healthy fats, protein, and micronutrients. They can be sprinkled on yogurt, added to smoothies, or

enjoyed as snacks.

Dairy-Free Alternatives Rich in Nutrients

- Almond Milk: Bursting with nutty flavor, almond milk is a popular dairy-free alternative. Fortified versions provide calcium, vitamin D, and vitamin B12, which are important for bone health and overall well-being.
- Coconut Yogurt: Made from coconut milk, this dairy-free yogurt offers healthy fats and a creamy texture. Bursting with probiotics, it supports gut health and provides a burst of flavor to breakfasts and snacks.
- Cashew Cheese: Cashew-based cheeses burst forth as a versatile dairy-free alternative. They can be used as spreads, dips, or toppings, providing a burst of creaminess and flavor.

Complete Meatless Meals for Balanced Nutrition

- Chickpea Stir-Fry: Sauté chickpeas with a burst of colorful vegetables like bell peppers, carrots, and broccoli. Bursting with protein and fiber, this stir-fry can be seasoned with herbs and spices for added flavor.
- Mushroom and Spinach Risotto: Prepare a creamy risotto bursting with umami flavors by using mushrooms and spinach. Arborio rice provides a burst of carbohydrates, and nutritional yeast can be added for a cheesy taste.
- Lentil and Vegetable Curry: Create a burst of exotic flavors by preparing a lentil and vegetable curry. Bursting with spices and aromatics, this dish

provides protein, fiber, and a medley of nutrients.

- Black Bean Burger: Make homemade black bean burgers bursting with protein, fiber, and flavor. Serve them on whole wheat buns with fresh veggies for a balanced and satisfying meal.

In conclusion, adopting a plant-based diet for liver health involves exploring a burst of nutrient-rich ingredients. Plant-based protein sources like legumes, tofu, and quinoa provide essential amino acids and other beneficial nutrients. Dairy-free alternatives like almond milk and coconut yogurt offer a burst of nutrients without relying on dairy. Complete meatless meals, whether stir-fries, risottos, curries, or burgers, burst forth with flavors and nutrients for balanced nutrition. By incorporating these plant-powered options, individuals can unravel the complexities of supporting liver health while enjoying a diverse and delicious range of meals.

CHAPTER SEVEN

Flavorful Herbs, Spices, and Sauces
Incorporating Turmeric, Garlic, Ginger, and More

Incorporating liver-supportive ingredients like turmeric, garlic, and ginger into your diet can be a burst of flavor and health benefits. These ingredients burst forth with anti-inflammatory, antioxidant, and detoxifying properties, making them valuable additions to your meals.

- Turmeric Golden Milk: Create a soothing and aromatic turmeric golden milk by simmering almond milk, turmeric, ginger, a touch of black pepper, and a hint of cinnamon. Bursting with anti-inflammatory compounds, this beverage supports liver health and provides comfort.
- Garlic-Roasted Vegetables: Enhance the flavor of roasted vegetables by tossing them with minced garlic and a burst of olive oil before baking. Garlic supports liver detoxification and adds a burst of savory taste to your dishes.
- Ginger-Lemon Dressing: Blend fresh ginger, lemon juice, olive oil, a touch of honey, and a sprinkle of salt to create a burst of zesty dressing for salads or grain bowls. Ginger's anti-inflammatory properties pair well with the burst of citrus.
- Turmeric Quinoa: Add ground turmeric to your

cooking water when preparing quinoa. The earthy flavor of turmeric complements the nuttiness of quinoa, bursting with color and health benefits.

Homemade Vinaigrettes and Sauces Without Added Sugars

Creating homemade vinaigrettes and sauces bursting with flavor and nutrients is a simple way to support liver health while avoiding added sugars.

- Balsamic Vinaigrette: Whisk together balsamic vinegar, Dijon mustard, minced garlic, a touch of honey or maple syrup (optional), and extra-virgin olive oil. This burst of flavor complements salads without the need for added sugars.
- Herb-Infused Olive Oil: Create your own herb-infused olive oil by infusing extra-virgin olive oil with fresh herbs like rosemary, thyme, or basil. Bursting with aromatic flavors, this oil can be drizzled over salads, grilled vegetables, or pasta.
- Tahini Dressing: Mix tahini, lemon juice, minced garlic, a touch of water, and a pinch of salt to create a creamy and flavorful dressing. Bursting with Middle Eastern flavors, this dressing pairs well with salads and roasted vegetables.
- Tomato and Roasted Red Pepper Sauce: Blend roasted red peppers, tomatoes, olive oil, a burst of garlic, and a touch of dried oregano to create a versatile sauce bursting with antioxidants. Use it as a pasta sauce or a dip for whole grain bread.

In conclusion, incorporating liver-supportive ingredients like turmeric, garlic, and ginger can be a burst of both flavor and health benefits in your meals. Creating homemade vinaigrettes and sauces without added sugars adds to the burst of creativity in your culinary endeavors. By infusing your dishes with these burst-worthy ingredients, you can demystify the complexities of supporting liver health while enjoying a diverse and flavorful range of foods.

CHAPTER EIGHT
Healthy Desserts to Satisfy Your Sweet Tooth

FRUIT-BASED TREATS

Satisfying your sweet cravings with fruit-based treats bursts forth as a healthier option that supports liver health. These treats provide natural sugars, fiber, and a burst of vitamins and antioxidants.

- Fruit Salad with Mint: Create a colorful burst of flavors by combining a variety of fresh fruits like berries, kiwi, oranges, and grapes. Top with chopped mint for a burst of freshness.
- Frozen Banana Bites: Slice bananas into bite-sized pieces, dip them in melted dark chocolate, and freeze until solid. Bursting with sweetness and a hint of bitterness from dark chocolate, these bites offer a satisfying treat.
- Baked Apples: Core apples and fill the center with a mixture of chopped nuts, cinnamon, and a drizzle of honey. Bursting with warm flavors, baked apples offer a healthier take on a classic dessert.

Low-Sugar Baked Goods

Enjoying baked goods bursting with flavor and goodness without excessive added sugars is a delightful way to support liver health.

- Oatmeal Raisin Cookies: Prepare oatmeal cookies

using whole grain oats, raisins, chopped nuts, and a touch of cinnamon. Bursting with natural sweetness, these cookies offer fiber and nutrients.

- Zucchini Bread: Bake zucchini into a burst of moist bread by using whole wheat flour, grated zucchini, unsweetened applesauce, and a hint of cinnamon. Bursting with veggies, this bread is a healthier option.
- Blueberry Muffins: Create burst-worthy blueberry muffins by using whole wheat flour, fresh or frozen blueberries, Greek yogurt, and a touch of honey for sweetness.

Nutrient-Dense Puddings and Yogurt Parfaits

Creating nutrient-dense puddings and yogurt parfaits bursting with flavors is a delightful way to incorporate beneficial ingredients.

- Chia Seed Pudding: Mix chia seeds with almond milk, a touch of vanilla extract, and a hint of honey. Let it sit overnight to create a burst of creamy chia seed pudding that's rich in fiber and omega-3 fatty acids.
- Yogurt Parfait: Layer Greek yogurt with a burst of mixed berries, chopped nuts, and a sprinkle of granola. Bursting with protein, probiotics, and antioxidants, this parfait is a well-rounded treat.
- Avocado Chocolate Pudding: Blend ripe avocado with unsweetened cocoa powder, a touch of honey, and a dash of almond milk to create a creamy and decadent chocolate pudding. Bursting with healthy fats and antioxidants, this pudding is a guilt-free indulgence.

In conclusion, indulging in fruit-based treats, low-sugar baked goods, and nutrient-dense puddings and yogurt parfaits can be a burst of enjoyment while supporting liver health. These treats offer creative ways to enjoy the sweetness of life without compromising on nutrition. By incorporating these burst-worthy options into your diet, you can demystify the complexities of supporting liver health while satisfying your taste buds.

CHAPTER NINE

Beverages for Liver Support
Hydration and Its Role in Liver Health

Hydration is a vital aspect of supporting liver health and overall well-being. The liver plays a significant role in detoxification, and proper hydration is essential for its optimal function. Adequate hydration helps the liver efficiently process toxins and waste products, preventing their buildup and potential damage. Bursting with importance, staying hydrated also supports digestion, circulation, and nutrient transport, contributing to overall liver health.

Herbal Teas and Infused Water Recipes

Incorporating herbal teas and infused water recipes can be a burst of hydration while adding a touch of flavor and health benefits.

Herbal Teas:

- Dandelion Root Tea: Bursting with liver-supportive properties, dandelion root tea aids in detoxification and digestion. Steep dried dandelion root in hot water for a soothing and beneficial beverage.
- Milk Thistle Tea: Bursting with antioxidants, milk

thistle tea supports liver health by protecting against oxidative stress. Choose a high-quality milk thistle tea for maximum benefits.

- Peppermint Tea: Peppermint tea bursts with a refreshing flavor and helps relax the digestive tract. It can support digestion, indirectly benefiting liver function.

Infused Water Recipes:

- Citrus Burst: Slice oranges, lemons, and limes and add them to a pitcher of water. Bursting with vitamin C and antioxidants, this infused water provides a refreshing burst of hydration.
- Cucumber-Mint Refresher: Combine cucumber slices and fresh mint leaves in water for a burst of cooling hydration. Mint adds a burst of freshness, and cucumber is known for its hydration benefits.
- Berry Burst: Mix a handful of fresh or frozen berries like strawberries, blueberries, and raspberries in water. Bursting with natural sweetness and antioxidants, this infused water is a delicious and hydrating option.

Reducing or Eliminating Sugary Drinks and Alcohol

Minimizing or eliminating sugary drinks and alcohol is pivotal for supporting liver health and overall well-being.

- Sugary Drinks: Bursting with added sugars, sodas, energy drinks, and sugary juices contribute to weight gain, insulin resistance, and fatty liver disease. Opt for water, herbal teas, and naturally flavored infused water to stay hydrated without added sugars.

- Alcohol: While moderate alcohol consumption might not be harmful to everyone, it's essential to limit alcohol intake to support liver health. Excessive alcohol consumption can lead to liver inflammation, fatty liver disease, and more severe liver conditions. Bursting with potential harm, reducing or eliminating alcohol is a step towards better liver health.

In conclusion, understanding the role of hydration in liver health is a burst of wisdom that contributes to overall well-being. Incorporating herbal teas and infused water recipes provides a creative way to stay hydrated while benefiting from the nutrients and antioxidants they offer. Reducing or eliminating sugary drinks and alcohol is pivotal for supporting liver health and preventing potential damage. By prioritizing hydration and making mindful beverage choices, you can demystify the complexities of supporting liver health while enjoying a burst of refreshment and nourishment.

CHAPTER TEN

Meal Planning and Portion Control
Creating Balanced Meal Plans

Crafting balanced meal plans bursting with nutrients and flavor is essential for managing fatty liver and overall health. Here's a burst of guidance to help you design well-rounded meal plans:

- Incorporate a Variety of Foods: Burst forth with a range of fruits, vegetables, whole grains, lean proteins, and healthy fats. This burst of variety ensures you're getting a spectrum of nutrients.
- Protein-Rich Choices: Include lean protein sources like poultry, fish, tofu, legumes, and nuts. Protein supports muscle health, balances blood sugar levels, and provides a sense of satiety.
- Complex Carbohydrates: Choose whole grains like brown rice, quinoa, and whole wheat bread for a burst of complex carbohydrates. These provide sustained energy and fiber.
- Healthy Fats: Include sources of healthy fats such as avocados, nuts, seeds, and olive oil. These fats burst with omega-3 fatty acids and antioxidants that support liver health.
- Portion Control: Bursting with importance, proper portion sizes prevent overeating and contribute to weight management. Balance your

plate with appropriate portions of protein, vegetables, and carbohydrates.

Proper Portion Sizes for Weight Management

Understanding portion sizes is pivotal for weight management and supporting liver health. Here's a burst of tips to guide you:

- Use Visual Cues: Bursting with simplicity, use your hand as a guide. A palm-sized portion of protein, a fist-sized portion of carbohydrates, and two handfuls of vegetables create a balanced plate.
- Read Labels: Bursting with information, read food labels to understand serving sizes. Pay attention to the number of servings in a package to avoid overeating.
- Practice Mindful Eating: Burst forth with mindfulness while eating. Pay attention to hunger and fullness cues, and eat slowly to allow your body to register satisfaction.
- Prevent Overloading: Bursting with wisdom, avoid overloading your plate with large portions. Start with smaller servings and listen to your body's signals.

Tips for Eating Out While Maintaining a Fatty Liver-Friendly Diet

Eating out can be a burst of enjoyment while maintaining a fatty liver-friendly diet. Follow these tips for a balanced and mindful experience:

- Check the Menu Ahead: Bursting with information, review the menu online before going out. This gives you time to make healthier choices and plan your meal.

- Choose Grilled or Steamed Options: Opt for grilled, baked, or steamed dishes instead of fried options. This burst of choice reduces unhealthy fats and calories.
- Request Modifications: Don't hesitate to burst forth with requests for modifications. Ask for dressings on the side, vegetables instead of fries, or whole grain options.
- Control Portions: Consider sharing a dish with a friend or asking for a to-go container to pack half of your meal before you start eating.
- Stay Hydrated: Bursting with importance, drink water throughout the meal. Staying hydrated helps control appetite and supports digestion.

In conclusion, creating balanced meal plans is a burst of strategy for managing fatty liver and overall health. Proper portion sizes contribute to weight management and prevent overeating. When eating out, following tips for making healthier choices and controlling portions ensures you can still enjoy dining while maintaining a fatty liver-friendly diet. By incorporating these strategies, you can demystify the complexities of managing fatty liver disease while enjoying flavorful and nourishing meals.

CHAPTER ELEVEN

Lifestyle Changes for Enhanced Liver Wellbeing
Importance of Regular Exercise

Regular exercise bursts forth as a powerful tool in promoting liver health and overall well-being. Exercise contributes to managing fatty liver disease by helping with weight management, improving insulin sensitivity, and enhancing overall cardiovascular health. Bursting with benefits, exercise also aids in reducing inflammation, which is a key factor in liver health.

- Weight Management: Bursting with significance, regular physical activity helps manage body weight. Maintaining a healthy weight reduces the risk of fatty liver disease and supports optimal liver function.
- Improved Insulin Sensitivity: Exercise enhances insulin sensitivity, which is crucial for preventing and managing conditions like insulin resistance and type 2 diabetes. Improved insulin sensitivity directly impacts liver health.
- Reduced Inflammation: Physical activity bursts forth with the ability to reduce chronic inflammation in the body. This is essential for maintaining liver health, as inflammation plays a role in the progression of liver diseases.
- Enhanced Blood Circulation: Bursting with

vitality, exercise promotes proper blood circulation. This supports the liver's detoxification process by efficiently transporting waste products and toxins out of the body.

Stress Reduction Techniques

Managing stress is pivotal for supporting liver health, as chronic stress can contribute to inflammation and worsen liver conditions. Bursting with benefits, incorporating stress reduction techniques can have a positive impact on your liver and overall well-being.

- Mindfulness Meditation: Burst forth with mindfulness meditation to reduce stress. Focusing on the present moment and practicing deep breathing can calm the nervous system and promote relaxation.
- Yoga: Bursting with flexibility and relaxation, yoga combines movement and breath to reduce stress and promote a sense of well-being.
- Deep Breathing Exercises: Practicing deep breathing techniques, such as diaphragmatic breathing, can trigger the body's relaxation response and help reduce stress.
- Nature Walks: Bursting with simplicity, spending time in nature can be a natural stress reliever. Nature walks provide a break from daily stressors and promote relaxation.

Getting Quality Sleep and Its Impact on Liver Function

Quality sleep is a burst of rejuvenation that profoundly affects liver function and overall health. During sleep, the body undergoes important processes, including cell repair, hormone regulation, and detoxification. Bursting with significance, sleep impacts liver health in various ways:

- Cell Repair and Regeneration: During deep sleep, the body repairs and regenerates cells. This burst of cellular repair supports the liver's ability to detoxify and function optimally.
- Hormone Regulation: Sleep plays a role in hormone regulation, including those that influence appetite, metabolism, and insulin sensitivity. Proper hormone balance supports liver health and overall well-being.
- Detoxification: The liver works to detoxify the body during sleep, removing waste products and toxins. Adequate sleep is pivotal for this essential burst of detoxification.
- Inflammation Reduction: Quality sleep helps regulate the body's immune response and reduces inflammation. Adequate sleep contributes to maintaining a healthy balance and reducing the risk of liver inflammation.

In conclusion, the importance of regular exercise bursts forth as a crucial component of supporting liver health and overall well-being. Stress reduction techniques contribute to a healthier liver by minimizing inflammation and promoting relaxation. Getting quality sleep is a burst of rejuvenation that positively impacts liver function, hormone regulation, and detoxification. By prioritizing these aspects of a healthy lifestyle, you can demystify the complexities of supporting liver health and enjoy a burst of vitality and balance.

CHAPTER TWELVE

Guidance for Long-Term Success
Monitoring Progress and Seeking Medical Advice

Monitoring your progress on the journey to liver health is a burst of accountability and awareness. Regular check-ins can help you understand how your lifestyle changes are affecting your liver function and overall well-being. Bursting with significance, consider the following steps:

- Regular Check-ups: Schedule regular medical check-ups to monitor your liver health and overall progress. Blood tests and imaging studies can provide valuable insights into the condition of your liver.
- Keep a Journal: Burst forth with a journal to track your dietary habits, exercise routine, stress levels, and sleep patterns. This burst of self-awareness can help you identify patterns and make necessary adjustments.
- Consult a Healthcare Professional: If you experience any unusual symptoms or changes in your health, seek medical advice promptly. Consulting a healthcare professional ensures you receive the appropriate guidance and care.

Adapting the Diet as Needed

Adapting your diet bursts forth as a dynamic process that

allows you to tailor your eating habits to your changing needs and goals. As you progress in your journey to liver health, consider these burst-worthy tips:

- Listen to Your Body: Pay attention to how your body responds to different foods and dietary changes. This burst of awareness can help you identify foods that support your liver health and those that may need adjustment.
- Gradual Changes: Bursting with wisdom, make dietary changes gradually. This approach allows your body to adjust and minimizes the risk of feeling overwhelmed.
- Consult a Nutritionist: Seeking guidance from a registered dietitian or nutritionist can provide personalized advice tailored to your needs and goals. They can help you adapt your diet in a way that supports your liver health journey.

Inspiring Success Stories and Testimonials

Drawing inspiration from success stories and testimonials can be a burst of motivation on your journey to liver health. Many individuals have successfully managed fatty liver disease through lifestyle changes. Reading about their experiences can provide valuable insights and encouragement.

- Online Communities: Bursting with camaraderie, join online communities or forums where individuals share their success stories and tips for managing fatty liver disease. These platforms can offer a burst of support and inspiration.
- Books and Resources: Look for books, articles, and resources written by experts or individuals

who have successfully improved their liver health. Bursting with knowledge, these resources can provide guidance and inspiration.

- Consult a Support Group: Consider joining a local support group or attending workshops focused on liver health. These gatherings provide an opportunity to connect with others who are on a similar journey and share their experiences.

In conclusion, monitoring your progress and seeking medical advice, adapting your diet as needed, and drawing inspiration from success stories are all bursts of empowerment on your journey to liver health. By staying informed, seeking support, and making adjustments when necessary, you can demystify the complexities of managing fatty liver disease and achieve your health goals.

CHAPTER THIRTEEN

Sample meal plan

Sample Meal Plans

Creating sample meal plans is a burst of guidance that helps you visualize how to incorporate balanced meals into your routine. Here are two sample meal plans for a day:

Sample Meal Plan 1:

Breakfast:

- Oatmeal topped with sliced bananas, chopped walnuts, and a sprinkle of cinnamon
- Herbal tea or water

Lunch:

- Grilled chicken salad with mixed greens, cherry tomatoes, cucumber, red onion, and a homemade balsamic vinaigrette
- Whole grain roll
- Infused water with lemon and mint

Snack:

- Greek yogurt with a handful of mixed berries and a drizzle of honey

Dinner:

- Baked salmon with a side of quinoa and steamed broccoli
- Side salad with mixed greens and a ginger-lemon

> dressing
> * Herbal tea or water

Sample Meal Plan 2:

Breakfast:

* Scrambled eggs with sautéed spinach, tomatoes, and a sprinkle of feta cheese
* Whole grain toast
* Herbal tea or water

Lunch:

* Lentil and vegetable curry with brown rice
* Side salad with mixed greens and a tahini dressing
* Infused water with cucumber and lime

Snack:

* Carrot and celery sticks with hummus

Dinner:

* Grilled tofu and vegetable stir-fry with a ginger-soy sauce
* Quinoa
* Herbal tea or water

In conclusion, providing nutritional information for recipes is a burst of transparency that empowers you to make informed dietary choices. Sample meal plans offer a burst of inspiration and guidance on how to structure balanced meals throughout the day. By incorporating nutritional information and sample meal plans into your routine, you can demystify the complexities of managing fatty liver disease and enjoy a burst of nourishing and flavorful meals.

CONCLUSION

In closing, this Fatty Liver Diet Cookbook bursts forth as a comprehensive guide to not only demystify the complexities of managing fatty liver disease but also to empower you with practical tools for vibrant well-being. Throughout these pages, we've embarked on a journey filled with burst-worthy flavors, nourishing ingredients, and evidence-based strategies that harmoniously support liver health.

From understanding the nuances of fatty liver disease to crafting nutrient-rich meals that burst with creativity and taste, we've explored a myriad of approaches to nourish both body and soul. Through the principles of balanced nutrition, the infusion of wholesome ingredients, and the adoption of mindful practices, you've gained the knowledge and tools to make informed choices that resonate with your health goals.

As you embark on this culinary adventure, may each recipe be a burst of inspiration to create nourishing dishes that nurture your body and celebrate the joy of eating well. Remember, this cookbook is not just a collection of recipes; it's a burst of transformation, a testament to the potential of food to heal, support, and energize.

Whether you're savoring a nutrient-dense smoothie, crafting a plant-powered masterpiece, or finding solace in stress-reducing techniques, each page reflects our commitment to your well-being. The journey to better liver health is a dynamic path, and this cookbook is your trusted companion, a burst of wisdom and flavor that guides you every step of the way.

In the realm of health, every choice is a burst of empowerment. Every bite, a burst of nourishment. Every meal, a burst of transformation. With this cookbook in hand, you're equipped to embrace the burst-worthy potential of nourishing your liver, body, and spirit.

Here's to your health, your journey, and the vibrant bursts of flavor that await you on the path to well-being. Embrace each burst with curiosity, savor every moment of growth, and remember, your choices have the power to create a life that truly bursts with vitality and fulfillment.

9 7 9 8 8 5 8 4 1 8 6 8 9